Nutritious Vegetarian Single-Serving Diabetic Recipes

Emily Hanson

ISBN: 9798395245489

Also by Emily Hanson

Satisfying Single Serving Vegan Recipes

Simple Healthy Smoothies For The 5:2 Diet

Crisis In Care Homes: A Shocking View From The Inside

Stimulating Creative Activities For One Person To Do At Home

To the memory of my mother Mary

with much love

Acknowledgement

My grateful thanks to Santhamma Plamkoottathil, who generously gave me help and advice, drawn from her seven years' experience as a diabetes nurse

CONTENTS

Introduction

Diabetes is a rapidly growing health problem. It's known as a silent killer because people often don't recognize the early signs and it may be many years before serious symptoms appear. So it can wreak havoc with people's health before it's diagnosed and can cause far too many premature deaths.

Moreover, studies show that if you have close family members with diabetes you're much more likely to develop it. In my case, since my mother and both my brothers were diagnosed with this condition, there's a clear genetic link.

Overweight, paying little attention to what I ate and hardly ever doing any exercise, I was certainly on that path. It wasn't until I was approaching middle age that I thought seriously about the distinct likelihood of getting diabetes myself.

Perhaps it was inevitable, I thought, that I would become diabetic in time. Yet, a small degree of research and a larger dose of common sense led me to conclude that I actually did have a choice in the matter. My predisposition to diabetes didn't mean that I simply needed to accept that developing the disease was a foregone conclusion that I could do nothing about. I could certainly rethink my lifestyle and begin to lead a healthier existence.

I decided to opt for a meat-free diet, resolved to walk the three mile journey to work, instead of driving, and set a regular bedtime for myself. Though I can't pretend that the changes I embarked on were easy. Nevertheless, my weight beginning to drop and friends' positive comments encouraged me to persevere. And, weighing less, I felt more inclined to exercise which, in its turn, improved my mood significantly.

However, the real wake-up call came two years ago, when, after a routine blood test, my husband was told that his elevated sugar level indicated that he was teetering on the brink of diabetes - he was prediabetic.

I began to intensively research diabetes with a view to not only improving both Andrew's health and my own, but also to providing my brothers with a better way forward to manage their condition than relying solely on medication to sort it.

The result is this book which begins with a simple explanation of the disease, why it develops, how it's treated and how to put yourself in control and prevent it taking over your life. That's followed by three weeks' worth of vegetarian breakfasts, lunches and dinners to vary as you wish. Maintaining the balance of carbohydrates, protein, fat, sodium, fibre and calories played an important part in coming up with these recipes.

A couple of years down the line Andrew is no longer classed at risk for diabetes as his blood sugar is back within the normal range.

Mark, one of my brothers, who was recently bereaved and now lives on his own, asked me to devise individual servings to simplify his life, so every meal in this book is for one person. Mark also happens to be vegetarian. Whether you already have diabetes, are trying to avoid becoming diabetic or are simply looking for plant-based meals to enable you to remain healthy, live longer and more enjoyably, I hope you enjoy mixing and matching the meals I have prepared for you.

Bon appétit!

An Overview of Diabetes

Definition

Diabetes is a condition where too much sugar is circulating in your blood.

Blood glucose, also known as blood sugar, is an essential source of energy that our cells use to keep our bodies in good working order. Insulin is a hormone produced by the pancreas to help the glucose from our food to reach the cells. When the pancreas doesn't produce insulin, produces too little or when it's not able to be used effectively by the body, the glucose stays in the blood, unable to get into the cells and be used.

Types of Diabetes

There are several different forms of diabetes with type 1, type 2 and gestational diabetes being the more common varieties.

Type 1 is where the pancreas is unable to produce any insulin to deal with glucose so it builds up in the bloodstream creating a high sugar level.

Type 2 occurs when either the pancreas makes insufficient insulin or when the insulin that it does produce doesn't work well enough to stop blood sugar levels from rising too high.

If a woman cannot make enough insulin during her

pregnancy she can develop high blood sugar. This is called gestational diabetes, is related specifically to the pregnancy and usually disappears when she has given birth.

Although looking briefly at these different manifestations of the disease, diabetes type 2 - the most common form - is the main focus of this book.

Causes of this Condition

Types 1, 2 and gestational diabetes all have a genetic link in that someone who has a close family member with a particular type of the disease has a greater chance of developing it.

Type 1 is considered to be an autoimmune response where the body mistakes the normal cells in the pancreas that are responsible for the production of insulin as foreign and destroys them.

Some of the hormones that get released during pregnancy increase a woman's need for more insulin to be made than usual. However, if her pancreas cannot meet this demand for extra insulin, her blood sugar rises too high and the results is gestational diabetes.

Research shows that the most probable cause for developing diabetes type 2 is being overweight. And, a sedentary lifestyle combined with a diet rich in fat and sugar is frequently responsible for obesity.

Potential Consequences

Without treatment diabetes is very likely, over time, to cause serious health issues, some of which can be fatal. Left unregulated, high levels of blood sugar can lead to poor circulation, skin and eye problems, nerve damage, heart disease, stroke, loss of kidney function... to name just some of the dreadful possibilities.

Prediabetes

If your blood sugar levels are outside the healthy range but not yet high enough to give a diagnosis of diabetes your GP will class you as prediabetic or borderline diabetic, which means that there is a significant likelihood, if no action is taken, that you will become diabetic. And, unfortunately, unless this is picked up in a blood test known as HbA1c, which reveals your average sugar level over the previous three months, you may well be unaware of this risk. With no obvious signs, it's unlikely that you'll know that you are in real danger of becoming very ill.

However, the good news is that knowledge is power. If you have been told that you are now prediabetic you are in a good position to do something about it. A diagnosis of diabetes in the future does not have to be a reality, it can be avoided.

Treating Diabetes

At this point in time there is no cure for diabetes. However, whichever type of this condition you have, it can be treated and carefully monitored to prevent any complications arising.

Once gestational diabetes is diagnosed, the pregnant woman is given a blood sugar meter and shown how to use it. She pricks her finger with a device called a lancet to put a drop of blood onto a test strip which is then measured by the meter to show her blood sugar level. Testing the level before and after meals enables her to track how well it's being controlled. Keeping a record of her blood sugar throughout the day enables her doctor to decide if she needs medication. Initially though, it's hoped that sticking to an agreed healthy eating plan and regular physical exercise will avoid the need for other interventions. She will be reviewed frequently.

To ensure that their sugar level is being kept under control, anyone with type 1 or 2 diabetes will see a diabetes nurse regularly. Their weight, cholesterol and blood pressure will also be measured.

Someone who has type 1 diabetes needs to be given insulin to manage their blood sugar. They administer this themselves either by injection or by using a pump which anticipates how much insulin is required and automatically delivers the correct dose.

Depending on the severity, a person with type 2 diabetes will be advised about making any necessary changes to their diet, physical activity, weight and general lifestyle, plus taking medication if it's deemed necessary. The aim with any form of diabetes is to keep blood sugar levels as close to normal as possible. Sometimes, the changes made are enough to bring blood sugar into normal parameters; this is called remission. So, although the diagnosis will always remain in place, to all intents and purposes, anyone who gets to and maintains this stage becomes virtually free of the disease.

 A diabetic may suffer from hyperglycaemia - when the level of sugar in blood is too high. Conversely, their blood sugar may be too low - hypoglycaemia. Both these occurrences can be stopped in their tracks with prompt treatment, good diabetes management and advice from a medical professional.

Diabetes & Diet

Initially, a diagnosis of diabetes can be worryingly confusing where diet is concerned. Eating is a pleasant activity for most of us. We are used to eating what we enjoy and meeting up with others for a meal and a chat. And, if you also have a sweet tooth, being told to avoid sugar in future may not feel doable. Yet, food high in sugar, can cause a sudden spike in blood glucose so, with the exception of the very occasional treat, it has to be seen as a pretty dangerous substance. However, although sugar is bad for you, consuming it causes the body to release dopamine - a feel good chemical - so you may have developed a craving for it; any changes made to your diet must be maintained for the rest of your life so they need to be realistic.

Luckily, most supermarkets now have many sugar-free products: jams, biscuits chocolate... and natural sweeteners to add to food, like stevia - derived from plants. Stevia is a really good option since it does not contain any sugar or calories and will not raise your blood glucose. It's also a lot sweeter than regular sugar so you only need to use a small amount.

It's not wise to use either saccharin or sucralose as both these artificial sweeteners have been found to cause blood glucose levels to rise.

Surprisingly, some brands of products, like bread and sauces do contain sugar so, until you get to know which ones don't, it's best to run your eye down the list of ingredients to check.

Eating regular, properly balanced meals is necessary for optimum health for any of us, diabetic or not. And, personally, I found that portion control was easier to achieve by investing in a set of smaller dinner plates.

Although salt doesn't affect blood sugar, it can increase blood pressure so keeping sodium to a minimum is also important for a healthy diet. You can do this by adding different herbs and spices to your meals.

Having diabetes means choosing foods with a low glycaemic index (or GI) which measures, on a scale of 0-100, how much the carbohydrates in food raise blood glucose level. I have used sweet potatoes in my recipes because their GI is lower than white potatoes. The net result is a slower conversion of the starch you've eaten into glucose in your blood, therefore the degree of fluctuation in your blood glucose after a meal will be lower. Sweet potatoes are nutritiously rich in fibre, potassium and vitamin A.

Oats, wholegrains, beans, pasta, lentils, most fruits and vegetables are examples of low GI foods and are all included in the recipes that follow.

Eating can remain a pleasurable activity. By adjusting your diet, by putting into your mouth food that is nutritious and healthy, your mood as well as your sugar level will improve. There's a great deal of truth in the saying 'You are what you eat'.

As with any medical condition, it's important to consult with your doctor/diabetes nurse before making any radical changes to your diet and lifestyle.

Going Forward

Having a genetic predisposition elevates your risk for diabetes type 2, as does being prediabetic. But if you opt for a healthy lifestyle it's possible to avoid developing it. And, if you already have the disease there's still much that you can do to slow down or even stop its progression.

Eating well, which means choosing foods that are lower in fat and fibre and eating more wholegrains, fruit and vegetables, is a sure-fire way of having more control over your health.

Deciding to exercise more each day - going for a brisk walk, swimming, dancing or cycling are all excellent choices; astonishingly, just eleven minutes a day is said to make a difference. The main thing is not to sit still for long periods of time.

Well thought out meals, moderate exercise and having good quality nights' sleep will contribute to a loss of any excess body weight, improve your overall physical and mental health and give you the best chance of living a longer, healthier, happier life.

Breakfasts

Scrambled Spicy Tofu on Toast

Ingredients

100g firm tofu

2 tsp rapeseed oil

1 small onion

1 medium clove garlic

¼ tsp turmeric

¼ tsp ground paprika

½ tsp ground cumin

1 small ripe vine tomato

1 heaped tsp freshly chopped parsley

1 slice wholemeal bread

Instructions

- Drain off excess liquid & mash tofu, in a bowl, using a fork
- Cut onion into thin slices

- Crush garlic or chop finely

- Dice tomato

- Heat oil gently in a frying pan

- Add onion slice & fry until softened, approx 5 min

- Add garlic & spices & cook for 1 min, stirring continuously

- Stir in tofu, increase heat to medium, tip tomato in, continue cooking until tomato softens, stirring frequently, approx 4 min

- Toast bread slice & transfer to serving plate

- Fold parsley into mixture & ladle onto toast

- Enjoy while hot

Nutty & Fruity Cottage Cheese

Ingredients

3 heaped tbsp cottage cheese

Pinch of ground cinnamon

1 level tbsp chopped pecan nuts

65g raspberries

Small pinch stevia

Instructions

- Scoop cottage cheese into a serving bowl & stir in cinnamon
- Sprinkle nuts over
- Top with raspberries & sprinkle with stevia

Deliciously Crunchy Fruity Toast

Ingredients

1 slice of whole grain brown bread

1 tbsp crunchy pure peanut butter

1 level tbsp fresh blueberries

2 large fresh strawberries, sliced

Instructions

- Toast bread slice
- Place toast on a small serving plate
- Spread peanut butter evenly over
- Top with blueberries & strawberry slices
- Savour each deliciously healthy bite!

Fibre-Filled Start to the Day

Ingredients

25g porridge oats

180ml unsweetened soya milk

¼ tsp vanilla extract

1 tsp chia seeds

Pinch of stevia, to taste

2 heaped tsp chopped almonds

75g fresh blueberries

1 tbsp low-fat natural Greek-style yogurt

Instructions

- Measure oats, soya milk, vanilla, chia seeds, stevia, 1 heaped tsp almonds & half the blueberries into a serving bowl & mix well
- Leave to stand for approx 20 min, then stir the mixture, adding a little more milk if the mixture is a bit dry

- Top with yogurt

- Sprinkle the rest of the almonds & blueberries over & your breakfast is ready to enjoy

Creamy Avocado & Kale Smoothie

Ingredients

1 small banana

½ ripe avocado

240ml unsweetened vanilla almond milk

65g chopped kale

1 level tbsp chia seeds

¼ tsp stevia, to taste

2 ice cubes

Instructions

- Slice banana & avocado
- Pour the milk into a blender
- Add banana & avocado slices
- Tip in kale, chia seeds, & stevia
- Pop in ice cubes & blitz until green & creamy
- Pour into a tall glass & drink thoughtfully

Nutty Peachy Ricotta on Toast

Ingredients

1 large slice of wholemeal bread

1 tbsp ricotta cheese

Pinch of cinnamon

1 tsp sugar-free fruit-based syrup

1 small sliced peach

1 tbsp chopped walnuts

Instructions

- Toast the bread
- While it's toasting, put cheese, cinnamon & syrup into a bowl & mix well
- Place toasted bread on a serving plate
- Scoop mixture from bowl onto toast
- Arrange peach slices over
- Sprinkle nuts on & enjoy every mouthful

Sweet Cherry Chocolate Oats

Ingredients

180ml unsweetened almond milk

28g porridge oats

1 tsp chia seeds

¼ tsp stevia

1 level tsp pure cocoa powder

¼ tsp grated coconut

¼ tsp grated dark chocolate

1 tbsp frozen cherries, thawed

1 tsp pure maple syrup

Instructions

- Pour almond milk into a small non-stick saucepan
- Stir in oats, chia seeds, stevia & cocoa
- Bring mixture to the boil, stirring frequently

- Reduce heat to low & simmer gently until oats are soft & almost all liquid is absorbed or until your desired consistency is reached

- Scoop porridge into a serving bowl

- Sprinkle with coconut & grated chocolate

- Scatter with cherries & drizzle maple syrup over to complete your sweet treat

Tasty Veg & Egg Bake

Ingredients

1 large vine tomato

¼ garlic clove

1 large mushroom

42g spinach

2 tsp extra virgin olive oil

1 medium free range egg

Pinch of freshly ground black pepper, to taste

1 tsp freshly chopped parsley

Instructions

- Preheat oven to 200^0C

- Cut tomato in half

- Chop garlic clove finely

- Slice mushrooms & spinach

- Dot tomato with garlic & place in an ovenproof dish

- Add mushroom slices

- Sprinkle with pepper & drizzle oil evenly over

- Bake for 10 min

- Meanwhile, put spinach into colander & pour boiling water over to wilt it

- Tip spinach onto a piece of kitchen towel, place another piece over & press to remove water

- Remove the dish from the oven & stir spinach into the other vegetables

- Create a space in the middle of the vegetables & break the egg into it

- Return dish to oven & continue baking for approx 8 min or until the egg is cooked to your satisfaction

- Transfer the bake onto a plate

- Garnish with parsley before serving

High Fibre Millet with Mandarin Oranges

Ingredients

28g millet

120ml unsweetened almond milk

60ml water

Small pinch of ground cardamom

Tiny pinch of stevia

½ tsp vanilla extract

Small pinch of cinnamon

Tiny pinch salt

56g tinned mandarin oranges, without juice

2 tsp flaked almonds

Instructions

- Put all ingredients except for mandarin oranges &
  almonds into a small lidded, non-stick saucepan

- Bring to the boil uncovered then reduce heat to low & cover

- Simmer, without stirring, for approx 20 minutes or until liquid is absorbed

- Stir in oranges then remove from heat

- Scoop mixture into a serving bowl

- Sprinkle almonds over before serving

Overnight Creamy Muesli

Ingredients

28g porridge oats

1 tsp dried goji berries

¼ tsp vanilla extract

200ml unsweetened almond milk

1 tsp ground flaxseed

1 tsp pumpkin seeds

1 tbsp natural yogurt

3 large freshly sliced strawberries

Instructions

- Put oats, goji berries, vanilla extract & almond milk into a serving bowl & stir well
- Cover & place in the fridge until morning
- Before serving for breakfast, stir in flaxseed & pumpkin seeds & top with yogurt & strawberries

Wholemeal Muffin with Topping

Ingredients

1 wholemeal muffin

1 tbsp pure peanut butter

1 small banana

2 small pinches of ground cinnamon

Instructions

- Cut muffin in half, toast both halves & place on a serving plate
- Spread each half evenly with peanut butter
- Slice banana & arrange slices equally on each muffin half
- Sprinkle each half with a pinch of cinnamon
- Enjoy!

Eggciting Breakfast

Ingredients

½ green bell pepper, deseeded

1 vine tomato

25g organic cucumber

2 fresh mint leaves

25g feta cheese

A squeeze of lemon

Pinch of freshly ground black pepper

1 cal olive oil spray

1 thick slice of wholemeal bread

1 large free range egg

Instructions

- Preheat grill

- Chop pepper, tomato, cucumber & mint & put into a
  bowl

- Crumble the feta cheese into the bowl & add a squeeze of lemon & black pepper

- Stir contents well

- Toast bread on one side only, remove from grill & place on a cutting board

- Use a glass tumbler to cut out a circle from the middle of the toast

- Toast the other side of the bread circle under grill & set aside for serving

- Lightly spray a non-stick frying pan with oil & heat

- Place bread slice, toasted side up in pan & crack egg into the circle

- Cook until egg has set, approx 2 min

- Meanwhile, place toasted bread circle in centre of a serving plate

- Use a spatula to transfer toast with egg onto the plate to cover the toasted circle

- Scoop mixture from bowl around the edge of the plate before serving

Wholegrain Toast with Cheesy Mushrooms

Ingredients

2 tsp rapeseed oil

84g button mushrooms

2 tbsp semi-skimmed milk

¼ tsp wholegrain mustard

4 tsp reduced fat cream cheese

1 medium slice wholegrain bread

1 level tbsp chopped chives

Instructions

- Wipe mushrooms using damp paper towel, then slice them
- Heat oil in non-stick frying pan on medium-high heat
- When oil is hot, add mushrooms & sauté for 4-5 min
- Meanwhile, toast bread slice, place on a serving plate & spread with 2 tsp cream cheese

- Add milk, mustard & 2 tsp of cream cheese to the mushrooms & stir until they are thoroughly coated
- Scoop cheesy mushroom mixture onto the toast & sprinkle with chives

Spicy Quinoa

Ingredients

60ml water

60ml apple juice

60g red & white quinoa

1 tsp grated ginger root

60ml unsweetened almond milk

2 tsp mixed chopped nuts

1 tsp chopped dried apricots

Small pinch stevia (optional)

2 tsp natural, fat-free yogurt

Instructions

- Bring water & apple juice to boil in a small non-stick saucepan on medium heat
- Meanwhile, rinse quinoa in a fine sieve under running cold water for 30 sec

- Add quinoa & ginger to pan, cover & reduce heat to low

- Simmer very gently for 15 minutes, stirring frequently

- Stir in almond milk & bring mixture to the boil, then remove pan from the heat. Allow to stand for 5 min

- Scoop into a bowl & sprinkle with nuts, apricots & stevia (if using)

Top with yogurt before serving

Sweet Potato & Veg Omelette with Herbs

Ingredients

2 tsp rapeseed oil

3 tbsp frozen mixed veg

2 large free range eggs

1 tbsp skimmed milk

Pinch of freshly ground black pepper

½ tsp dried oregano

1 tsp freshly chopped basil

80g cooked sweet potato, chopped into small chunks

Instructions

- Heat oil in a non-stick frying pan over medium heat
- Stir in mixed veg & sauté until softened
- Break eggs into a bowl, add milk & whisk well
- Mix pepper, oregano & basil into the egg mixture
- Add sweet potato chunks to the sautéed veg
- Pour egg mixture evenly over contents in frying pan

- Reduce heat & cook until the egg is set

- Transfer your omelette to a serving plate

Creamy Spiced Oats

Ingredients

180ml unsweetened almond milk

28g porridge oats

1 tsp ground flaxseed

¼ tsp ground turmeric

Pinch of ground cinnamon

35g cottage cheese

1 tbsp fresh blueberries

Instructions

- Pour almond milk into a small non-stick saucepan & bring to the boil
- Turn heat to low & stir in oats
- Simmer gently for approx 4-5 min until creamy, stirring frequently
- Remove from heat & stir in flaxseed, turmeric, cinnamon & cottage cheese

- Spoon into a serving bowl & top with blueberries

Tomatoes, Courgettes & Egg

Ingredients

200g courgettes

100g cherry tomatoes, halved

2 tsp rapeseed oil

1 small crushed garlic clove

Pinch of freshly ground black pepper

1 free range egg

4 fresh basil leaves, torn

Small wholegrain roll

Instructions

- Cut courgettes into small chunks & tomatoes into halves
- Heat oil in a non-stick lidded frying pan
- Put courgettes into the pan & fry for approx 5 min or until softened, turning frequently

- Add tomatoes & garlic & pepper & cook for a further 3 min

- Create a gap in the centre of the mixture, break egg into it, cover & cook until it's just as you like it

- Transfer to a serving plate, garnish with basil & serve, while hot, with the roll

Sweet Potatoes with Spring Onions & Mushrooms

Ingredients

1 tbsp rapeseed oil

75g boiled sweet potatoes, cut into large chunks

3 trimmed & sliced spring onions

75g button mushrooms, cut into halves

½ tsp plain wholemeal flour

75ml semi-skimmed milk

15g grated mature cheddar cheese

Pinch of freshly ground black pepper

Instructions

- Put oil into a non-stick frying pan on medium-high heat
- Add potatoes, mushrooms & spring onions & sauté for 4- 5 min or until mushrooms & onions are soft
- Add flour & stir well before slowly adding milk, stirring continuously

- Stir in the cheese & season with pepper

- Ladle mixture onto a serving plate & it's ready to eat

43

Speedy, Spiced Carrot Cake

Ingredients

1 small carrot

2 level tbsp self raising wholemeal flour

1 level tsp pure maple syrup

½ tsp ground mixed spice

Pinch of ground cinnamon

1 large free range egg

2 tbsp unsweetened almond milk

2 tsp natural fat-free yogurt

Instructions

- Peel & grate carrot
- Put flour, maple syrup, mixed spice & cinnamon into a bowl & stir well
- Break egg into a small bowl & beat then add to the flour mixture & stir vigorously
- Stir in half the grated carrot & all the almond milk

- Spoon into a microwavable mug & cook in the microwave on a high setting or until mixture has risen, approx 1 min depending on wattage
- Take out the mug & allow to stand for 2 min Top with yogurt & sprinkle on the rest of the carrot before serving

Hearty Oats, Seeds & Nuts

Ingredients

28g porridge oats

1 level tbsp chia seeds

60ml water

180ml semi-skimmed milk

1 tbsp raspberries

½ tsp dried cranberries

1 tbsp blackberries

1 heaped tsp chopped mixed nuts

1 tbsp fat-free natural yogurt

1 tsp pure maple syrup

2 chopped mint leaves

Instructions

- Put oats, chia seeds, water & milk in a saucepan, stir & bring to the boil over medium heat

- Turn heat to low & simmer contents until they reach your desired consistency, approx 4-5 min
- Scoop mixture into a serving bowl & sprinkle with nuts
- Spoon on the berries & drizzle with maple syrup

Smooth Pear & Ginger

Ingredients

120ml unsweetened almond milk

168g ripe pears, chopped

¼ tsp ground ginger

2 ice cubes

Instructions

- Pour almond milk into a blender
- Pop in the chopped pears
- Add ginger & ice cubes
- Whizz thoroughly until smooth
- Pour into a glass & sip slowly

Lunches

Warming Basil & Tomato Soup

Ingredients

1 tablespoon olive oil spread

56g chopped onions

1 minced medium clove garlic

¼ tsp dried basil

¼ tsp paprika

Small pinch chilli powder

Small pinch freshly ground sea salt

120ml low salt vegetable stock

400g can chopped tomatoes

1 tsp freshly chopped basil

Instructions

- Melt olive oil spread in a saucepan over medium heat
- Tip in onions & cook until softened, approx 1 min, stirring continuously
- Add garlic, dried basil, paprika, chilli powder & salt & stir another min

- Stir in vegetable stock & canned tomatoes, including juice
- When mixture reaches boiling point, lower heat & simmer for 20 min, stirring every so often
- Allow soup to cool slightly before transferring to a blender & whizzing to the consistency you want
- If necessary return soup to pan to reheat
  Pour into a bowl & garnish with fresh basil before serving

Easy Creamy Spaghetti

Ingredients

75g wholewheat spaghetti

Pinch of low sodium salt

1 tbsp olive oil spread

1 thinly sliced garlic clove

2 tbsp grated mozzarella cheese

Pinch of freshly ground black pepper

1 tbsp freshly chopped parsley

Instructions

- Boil a pan of water, with pinch of salt added, on high heat
- Add spaghetti & cook according to instructions on packet
- Drain pasta, reserving 2 tbsp of the water in a cup
- Tip spaghetti into a bowl
- Gently heat olive oil spread to melt, in the same saucepan used above

- Stir in garlic & cook until slightly browned, approx 1 min
- Remove from heat & scoop spaghetti into the saucepan, adding the reserved water
- Toss to thoroughly coat spaghetti with melted spread, stir in cheese & return it to the bowl

  Season with pepper & garnish with parsley to serve

Cheesy Onion & Mixed Peppers

Ingredients

112g cottage cheese

2 large spring onions

½ small green pepper

½ small orange pepper

½ small red pepper

Pinch of freshly ground black pepper

1 tsp freshly chopped basil

Instructions

- Put cottage cheese into a serving bowl
- Deseed & chop all the peppers
- Trim spring onions & & slice finely
- Stir onions & peppers into cottage cheese
- Sprinkle with ground pepper & garnish with basil

Wholegrain Toast with Spicy Avocado

Ingredients

1 thick slice of wholegrain bread

1 small avocado

A small wedge of lemon

Pinch of dried chilli flakes

Instructions

- Toast bread
- While it's toasting mash avocado
- Place toast on a serving plate & spread avocado evenly over
- Squeeze lemon juice over & sprinkle with chilli flakes

Quinoa with Wild Mushroom, Peas & Peppers

Ingredients

4 large lettuce leaves

250ml low sodium vegetable stock

25g dried porcini mushrooms

50g quinoa

85g sliced broccoli

½ green pepper, chopped

1 tsp capers

1 tbsp frozen peas

2 tsp tamari

2 tsp soy sauce

1 tsp freshly chopped basil

1 tsp smoked paprika

Instructions

- Tear lettuce leaves into small pieces & put into a small bowl
- Pour stock into a non-stick lidded saucepan & bring to the boil on high heat
- Add mushrooms, quinoa, broccoli, pepper, capers, peas, 1 tsp tamari & soy sauce, stir well until boiling, then reduce heat to low & cover
- Simmer for 8-10 min or until liquid is absorbed
- If quinoa is not yet fluffy, remove from heat, cover & allow to stand for a few min
- Spoon onto a serving plate, sprinkle with paprika & basil & drizzle rest of tamari over
- Serve with your bowl of lettuce

Mixed Roasted Vegetables

Ingredients

¼ cauliflower

1 small red onion

 1 medium carrot

5 Brussels sprouts

Pinch freshly ground black pepper

Small pinch sea salt

2 tsp extra virgin olive oil

1 tsp freshly chopped mint

1 tsp freshly chopped parsley

2 level tsp crushed walnuts

Instructions

- Heat oven to 180^0C

- Meanwhile, break cauliflowers into florets, slice onion finely, chop carrot into wedges & halve the sprouts

- Line a small baking tray with foil & spread vegetables onto it

- Sprinkle with pepper & salt

- Drizzle oil over all veg

- Roast in oven for approx 35 min or until vegetables are lightly browned

- Transfer vegetables to a serving plate
  Scatter mint & parsley over & sprinkle on the nuts before serving

Colour-Filled Salad

Ingredients

2 tsp extra virgin olive oil

1 tsp freshly squeezed lemon juice

½ tsp freshly chopped parsley

Pinch of freshly ground black pepper

Handful of lettuce

1 baby cucumber

½ small green pepper

½ small orange pepper

½ small onion

3 radishes

1 medium vine tomato

3 fresh mint leaves

Instructions

- Combine oil, lemon juice, parsley & pepper in a bowl to make the dressing
- Shred lettuce & arrange on a serving plate
- Slice cucumber, peppers, onion & radishes & dice tomato
- Sprinkle on dressing, toss well & place on bed of lettuce
- Decorate with mint leaves before serving

Stuffed Mushrooms

Ingredients

3 large mushrooms

½ tbsp red peppers, chopped

½ tbsp tomatoes, chopped

½ tbsp olives, chopped

1 small garlic clove

¼ t tbsp fresh parsley, finely chopped

¼ tsp freshly chopped oregano

Freshly ground black pepper, to taste

¼ tsp freshly squeezed lemon juice

28g crumbled feta cheese

1 tsp extra virgin olive oil

1 tsp freshly chopped parsley

Instructions

- Preheat oven to 190⁰C

- Clean mushrooms with damp paper towelling

- Remove stalks & hollow out the heads

- Line a baking tray with foil

- Put tomatoes, peppers, olives, parsley, oregano, pepper, lemon juice & feta cheese into a bowl

- Crush garlic into the mix, add olive oil & stir well until mixture is thoroughly coated

- Fill the mushroom heads equally & put them onto the baking tray

- Cook for approximately 20 min

- Serve on a plate & garnish with the parsley

Simple Lentil & Beetroot Soup

Ingredients

250g cooked beetroot

1 crushed garlic clove

1 small apple

250ml low sodium vegetable stock

100g of canned green lentils, drained

Pinch of freshly ground black pepper

1½ tsp black onion seeds

Instructions

- Chop beetroot into chunks
- Remove apple core & cut apple into slices
- Put beetroot, garlic, apple slices, stock, lentils, pepper & 1 tsp of the onion seeds into a blender
- Whizz to a smooth consistency
- Pour into a saucepan & heat slowly until hot

- Transfer soup to a bowl & sprinkle remaining ½ tsp onion seeds over to serve

Wholewheat Waffle with Peanut Butter & Berry Topping

Ingredients

1 wholewheat waffle

1 tbsp pure peanut butter

56g fresh raspberries & ripe strawberries

Tiny pinch of stevia (optional)

Instructions

- Toast waffle & slice in half
- Spread peanut butter evenly over both halves
- Put berries & stevia into a bowl & mash, using a fork
- Divide berry mixture, spreading equally onto waffle halves

Filled Pitta Bread

Ingredients

1 ready-to-fill wholemeal pitta bread

2 tbsp hummus

1 small vine tomato

½ orange pepper

 6 slices of organic cucumber

1 tbsp torn lettuce leaves

Instructions

- Spread hummus on half of inside of pitta bread
- Slice tomato & deseed & slice pepper
- Arrange tomato, pepper & cucumber slices on top of hummus
- Insert the lettuce
- Close bread & place on a serving plate, cut in half & it's ready to eat

Tofu, Chinese Style

Ingredients

75g uncooked brown basmati rice

4 tsp rapeseed oil

75g extra firm tofu

½ red bell pepper

½ onion

1 large clove garlic

1 heaped tsp tomato purée

80g pineapple chunks

1 tbsp organic apple cider vinegar

½ tbsp soy sauce

50ml water

1 heaped tsp sesame seeds

Instructions

- Cook rice according to instructions on packet

- Meanwhile, cut tofu & pepper into small chunks

- Slice onion into thin wedges & finely slice garlic

- Heat 2 tsp oil in non-stick frying pan on medium heat

- Stir in tofu & fry for 5 min or until golden brown, turning frequently

- Transfer tofu to a bowl & set to one side

- Put remaining 2 tsp oil into the frying pan on high & heat

- Add pepper, onion & garlic & cook until soft, approx 5 min

- Add tomato purée, pineapple, vinegar, soy sauce & water

- Simmer gently for 1 min to reduce liquid slightly

- Return tofu to the pan & stir briefly to reheat

- Drain rice & spoon into a serving bowl

- Top with tofu mixture & sprinkle sesame seeds over

Cauliflower & Spring Onion Soup

Ingredients

240ml low sodium vegetable stock

1 tbsp freshly squeezed lemon juice

½ medium head of cauliflower

2 tsp rapeseed oil

1 tbsp chopped spring onion

Pinch of ground nutmeg

¼ tsp freshly ground black pepper

Crusty wholemeal roll

Instructions

- Heat stock & lemon juice in a large saucepan to boiling point on high heat
- Break cauliflower into florets & add to saucepan
- Simmer until tender, approx 10 min
- Meanwhile, heat oil in a non-stick frying pan on medium heat

- Stir in spring onion & cook until soft, approx 5 min

- Stir spring onion into the pan containing cauliflower& stock

- Pour the soup into a blender

- Add nutmeg & pepper & purée until smooth

- Pour into serving bowl & enjoy with the roll

Quick Veggie Lunch

Ingredients

1 small courgette

1 small yellow pepper

½ medium onion

2 tsp rapeseed oil

1 ripe vine tomato

1 minced garlic clove

½ tsp Italian seasoning

Pinch of freshly ground black pepper

1 tbsp grated gruyère cheese

Instructions

- Slice courgettes & deseed & chop yellow pepper
- Cut onion into thin slices
- Heat oil in a non-stick frying pan on medium heat
- Stir in courgette, chopped pepper & onion

- Cook until veg is tender, approx 6-8 min, stirring
  frequently

- Chop tomato & add to pan together with garlic,
  seasoning & black pepper

- Continue cooking for 3 min, stirring frequently

- Remove from heat & scoop into a serving bowl

  Sprinkle with grated gruyère cheese to complete

Almond & Mixed Berry Smoothie

Ingredients

250ml unsweetened almond milk

1 small just ripe medium banana

1 tbsp chia seeds

110g frozen mixed berries

2 tsp almond butter

Instructions

- Pour milk into a blender
- Slice banana & put into blender
- Add chia seeds, berries & almond butter
- Blitz on high until all contents are combined
- Pour into a serving glass

Simply Sweet Cinnamon Potato

Ingredients

1 large sweet potato

4 tbsp natural fat-free yoghurt

2 level tsp ground cinnamon powder

Instructions

- Preheat oven to 200^{0}C
- Use a fork to pierce potato in several places
- Place potato on a foil-lined baking tray & bake in oven for 1 hr, testing with a sharp knife to make sure inside is soft
- Put potato onto a plate & cut in half lengthwise
- Spoon 2 tbsp of yoghurt onto each half
- Sprinkle each yoghurt topped potato half with 1tsp of cinnamon to serve

Eggs with Tomatoes Peppers & Onion

Ingredients

1 small red pepper

1 small onion

2 tsp rapeseed oil

 ½ tsp smoked paprika

½tsp dried chilli flakes

1 small crushed clove of garlic

¼ tsp cumin seeds

200g tinned chopped tomatoes

Pinch of freshly ground pepper

2 large free range eggs

1 heaped tbsp freshly chopped parsley

1 small crusty piece of wholemeal bread

Instructions

- Deseed & slice pepper

- Chop onion
- Heat oil in a non-stick frying pan on medium heat
- Add chopped pepper & onion to pan & sauté for approx 5 min until soft
- Lower heat, add paprika, chilli flakes, garlic & cumin seeds, season with ground pepper & stir well for 30 sec
- Stir in chopped tomatoes & simmer mixture for 4-5 min or until it starts to thicken
- Create 2 wells in the mixture & crack an egg into each well
- Simmer gently until eggs are cooked to the way you like them
- Carefully transfer the mixture to a serving plate & sprinkle parsley evenly over
- Enjoy with the crusty bread

Tempting Tofu Lunch

Ingredients

1 small courgette

1 medium tomato

1 clove of garlic

100g firm tofu

½ tsp ground cumin

½ tsp mustard powder

2 tsp rapeseed oil

112g sliced mushrooms

½ tsp low sodium soy sauce

50g spinach, rinsed & chopped

½ tsp lemon juice

Pinch of freshly ground black pepper

Instructions

- Chop courgette & cut tomato into small chunks

- Mince garlic

- Drain tofu & crumble it into a bowl

- Stir in cumin & mustard & mix well

- Heat olive oil in a non-stick lidded frying pan on medium heat

- Add garlic, courgette, tomato chunks, mushrooms & stir thoroughly

- Sauté for a couple of min

- Reduce heat before adding soy sauce, spinach, tofu, lemon juice & pepper

- Cover pan & continue cooking for about 5 min, until veg is soft, stirring frequently

- Scoop mixture onto a serving plate & enjoy while hot

Wholegrain Toast with Egg Cheese & Chives

Ingredients

2 medium slices wholegrain bread

1 medium free range egg

50g grated gruyère cheese

1 tsp freshly chopped chives

Pinch of cayenne pepper

Instructions

- Preheat oven to 200^{0}C
- Toast bread lightly
- Crack egg into a bowl & whisk well
- Stir in grated cheese & chives
- Place toast slices on a foil-lined baking tray
- Spread egg & cheese mixture evenly onto both pieces of toast right to the edges
- Sprinkle with cayenne pepper

- Bake in the oven until the cheese begins to bubble & turn slightly brown, approx 10 min

- Use a spatula to transfer toasts to a serving plate & enjoy your satisfying lunch

Speedy Salad

Ingredients

2 tsp extra virgin olive oil

Zest of ¼ lemon

Pinch of freshly ground black pepper

84g cherry tomatoes

½ tsp small red onion

4cm organic cucumber

168g drained tinned chickpeas, rinsed with cold water

4 large lettuce leaves

1 lemon wedge

Instructions

- Put oil, lemon zest & black pepper into a bowl & mix thoroughly
- Cut tomatoes into halves & add
- Chop onion finely & stir in
- Chop cucumber & add to bowl

- Mix contents of bowl well & allow to stand for a couple of min to infuse

- Add chickpeas & stir to coat completely

- Arrange lettuce leaves, on a serving plate, to form a bed

- Spoon contents of bowl onto the lettuce & squeeze lemon over

Chunky Veggie Soup

Ingredients

2 tsp rapeseed oil

50g chopped celery

1 medium carrot, peeled & chopped

28g chopped onions

1 clove garlic, minced

240ml low sodium vegetable broth

1 small sweet potato, peeled & chopped

1 tbsp sweetcorn

1 small tomato, chopped

28g green beans, chopped

Small pinch dried thyme

Pinch of freshly ground black pepper

Instructions

- Heat oil in a non-stick lidded saucepan

- Stir in celery, carrot & onion & cook gently for 3 min

- Add garlic & continue cooking for 1 min, stirring continuously

- Pour in broth & stir well

- Stir in remaining ingredients & bring to the boil

- Turn heat to low, cover & simmer gently for 20 min

- Ladle soup into a serving bowl

Sweet Potato & Peanut Korma

Ingredients

60g wholegrain basmati rice

2 tsp rapeseed oil

½ yellow pepper, chopped

20g diced onion

1 tsp korma curry paste

150g cooked sweet potato, cut into chunks

227g tinned chopped tomatoes

50ml water

½ vegetable stock cube

1 tsp pure smooth peanut butter

30g baby spinach leaves

Heaped tsp lightly salted chopped peanuts

Instructions

- Put oil in a saucepan over medium heat

- Stir in pepper & onion

- Cook for 5 min or until soft, stirring frequently

- Meanwhile, begin cooking basmati rice separately, according to instructions on packet

- Stir curry paste into pepper & onion, add potato chunks & tomatoes & stir for 1 min

- Add water, stock cube & peanut butter & continue stirring until just beginning to boil

- Reduce heat to low & simmer very gently for approx 10 min or until sauce thickens

- Chop spinach leaves

- Remove curried mixture from heat & stir in the spinach

- Transfer cooked rice to middle of a serving plate & scoop curry mix onto it

- Scatter peanuts over & serve while hot

Heartily Healthy Stew

Ingredients

2 tsp rapeseed oil

1 medium onion

75g mushrooms

1 crushed garlic clove

3 tbsp tomato paste

40g millet

80g dry red lentils

75g sweet potato

350ml water

1 tbsp freshly chopped parsley

Bowl of your choice of mixed salad

Instructions

- Slice onion

- Chop mushrooms

- Peel & dice sweet potato

- Heat oil in a non-stick lidded pan

- Add onion slices & fry on low heat until translucent, approx 5 min

- Add mushrooms & garlic & cook for 3 min, stirring continuously

- Stir in tomato paste, millet, lentils, sweet potato & water

- Cover & bring mixture to the boil on medium-high heat

- Reduce heat, cover & simmer for 15 min

- Ladle contents of pan onto a serving plate

- Garnish with parsley & serve with your bowl of salad

Pasta with Vegetables

Ingredients

1 medium-sized carrot

2 vine tomatoes

1 garlic clove

1 small courgette

1 small onion

56g broccoli florets

¼ tsp Italian seasoning

Small pinch of salt

Pinch of freshly ground black pepper

2 tsp extra virgin olive oil

56g uncooked wholewheat pasta spirals

1 tbsp olive oil spread

1 tbsp grated mozzarella cheese

Instructions

- Preheat oven to 220⁰C
- While it's heating, peel carrot & cut into long, thin slices
- Cut tomatoes into halves & chop garlic
- Cut courgette into wedges
- Slice onion & broccoli florets
- Place all vegetables on a foil-lined baking tray
- Sprinkle with Italian seasoning, salt & pepper
- Drizzle with oil & toss everything, to coat veg thoroughly
- Bake in oven until the vegetables are starting to brown, approx 20 min
- In the meantime, cook pasta according to instructions on packet
- Drain pasta & tip into a serving bowl
- Add olive oil spread & mix well
- Sprinkle with mozzarella cheese & enjoy straight away

Kidney Beans with Pepper, Aubergine & Squash

Ingredients

130g (drained weight) tinned red kidney beans

½ medium onion

1 garlic clove

½ orange pepper

75g butternut squash

½ aubergine

2 tsp rapeseed oil

2 tbsp tomato paste

Pinch of freshly ground black pepper

1 tbsp freshly chopped parsley

50g whole grain basmati rice

Instructions

- Rinse kidney beans in cold running water
- Slice onion, garlic, & pepper

- Dice squash & aubergine

- Heat oil in a lidded non-stick frying pan

- Sauté onion & garlic until onion is softening

- Add squash, aubergine, pepper & kidney beans

- Add tomato paste & ground pepper & stir well

- Pour in sufficient water to cover mixture

- Bring to the boil, stirring continuously

- Lower heat, cover & simmer for 15 min

- Meanwhile cook rice, following instructions on packet

- Spoon mixture in pan onto a serving plate & sprinkle with parsley

- Arrange cooked rice around mixture to serve

Warming Curried Chickpeas

Ingredients

75g of uncooked basmati rice

2 tsp rapeseed oil

56g chopped onion

Small pinch of ground ginger

1 minced garlic clove

1 tsp curry powder

Small pinch of salt

180ml tinned coconut milk

120ml low-sodium vegetable broth

Few drops of Tabasco sauce, to taste

2 tsp pure maple syrup

1 small tin chickpeas, drained & rinsed with cold water

Instructions

- Cook rice according to instructions on packet

- Heat oil in a non-stick frying pan on medium heat

- Stir in onion & sauté until it's softening

- Add ginger, curry powder, salt & garlic & cook for another min

- Stir in coconut milk, broth, Tabasco sauce & maple syrup & bring to the boil

- Stir in chickpeas, lower the heat & simmer the mixture, stirring frequently, for 8 -10 min or until sauce has thickened

- Spoon cooked rice onto a serving plate, making a space in the middle for the curry mixture

Saucy Broccoli & Cauliflower with Green Salad

Ingredients

½ small head of broccoli

½ small head of cauliflower

Small pinch of salt

Pinch of freshly ground black pepper

10g olive spread

10g plain wholemeal flour

1 tsp wholegrain mustard

125ml unsweetened almond milk

40g grated cheddar cheese

Bowl of green salad

Instructions

- Separate broccoli & cauliflower into small florets
- Slice broccoli & cauliflower stalks thinly
- Boil a saucepan of water & sprinkle in salt & pepper

- Add florets & stalks & boil until just tender, approx 4 min
- Drain veg, cover & put to one side in a warmed serving bowl
- Melt spread in a saucepan over a low heat & stir flour until a smooth mix is obtained
- Add mustard & pour milk in little by little, stirring continuously until the sauce thickens & is smooth (add a little more milk if it gets too thick)
- Add cheese & stir until it melts
- Remove sauce from heat & pour over broccoli & cauliflower
- Enjoy with the green salad

Creamy Penne Pasta

Ingredients

84g dry penne pasta

2 tsp rapeseed oil

1 spring onion

1 small minced garlic clove

35g soft goat's cheese

35g baby spinach

Small pinch of salt

Pinch of freshly ground black pepper

25g grated mozzarella cheese

1 tbsp chopped basil

Instructions

- Cook pasta following instructions on packet
- Trim & chop spring onion
- Heat oil on medium heat in a non-stick saucepan

- Add spring onion & cook until tender, approx 5 min

- Add garlic & cook for 1 more min

- Drain cooked pasta, keeping 120ml of the cooking water

- Pour the saved pasta water onto spring onion & garlic

- Add goat's cheese & stir continuously until cheese melts, approx 2 min, adding a little water to thin the sauce, if required

- Stir pasta & spinach into the sauce & cook briefly until spinach wilts

- Season with salt & pepper

- Scoop mixture into a serving bowl & sprinkle with mozzarella

- Finish by scattering basil over

Mushroom & Leek with Spiralised Veg

Ingredients

2 tsp rapeseed oil

1 thinly sliced small leek

1 finely sliced garlic clove

125g sliced mushrooms

Small pinch chilli flakes

1 level tsp dried oregano

1 tsp toasted pumpkin seeds

1tsp toasted sunflower seeds

1 medium carrot, spiralised

1 small courgette, spiralised

1 tbsp natural fat-free yogurt

Sprinkle freshly ground black pepper

1 tsp reduced fat grated Cheddar cheese

1 tsp freshly chopped basil

Instructions

- Heat oil in a non-stick pan
- Add leek & cook on low heat for 3 minutes, stirring frequently
- Stir in garlic, mushrooms, chilli & oregano
- Cook gently for 4 minutes, stirring regularly
- Put spiralised carrot & courgette into boiling water & leave for 2 min
- Transfer spiralised veg to a serving bowl
- Stir yogurt into mushroom mixture
- Spoon mushroom mixture onto spiralised veg
- Sprinkle with toasted seeds, black pepper, cheese & basil

Veggie Bolognese

Ingredients

½ small carrot

¼ stick of celery

½ small onion

2 tsp rapeseed oil

1 small crushed clove garlic

Pinch of dried chilli flakes

¼ tsp fennel seeds

100g passata

60g dried red lentils

200 ml water

1 small bay leaf

¼ teaspoon dried oregano

Pinch of freshly ground black pepper

75g wholewheat spaghetti

1 tbsp grated Emmental cheese

1 tbsp chopped fresh basil

Instructions

- Dice celery, carrot & onion

- Heat oil in a non-stick, lidded saucepan

- Add diced vegetables & fry, covered, on low heat until veg is soft, approx 3-4 min, stirring occasionally

- Stir in garlic, chilli flakes & fennel seeds & cook for 1min

- Rinse lentils under cold running water

- Add passata, lentils, water, bay leaf, oregano & black pepper & bring mixture to the boil

- Reduce heat to low, cover & simmer until lentils are cooked & sauce has thickened, approx 20 min, stirring often & adding a dash more water if mixture is too thick

- Meanwhile, cook pasta following instructions on the packet

- Once pasta is drained, return it to the saucepan it was cooked in & stir in the sauce

- Scoop into a bowl & garnish with the cheese & basil to serve

Easy Orzo Salad

Ingredients

56g wholewheat orzo pasta

28g red onion

28g sun-dried tomatoes

50g spinach leaves

28g toasted pine nuts

6 pitted Kalamata olives

 28g feta cheese

For Dressing

1tsp balsamic vinegar

2 tsp extra virgin olive oil

Pinch of freshly ground black pepper

Small pinch of dried basil

Instructions

- Cook orzo earlier in the day, following instructions on packet, drain & allow to stand until cold
- Chop onion, tomatoes & spinach
- Put onion, tomato, spinach, pine nuts & olives into a serving bowl
- Crumble in the feta cheese
- Add cold orzo & stir contents of bowl well

To Make Dressing

- Put vinegar, oil, black pepper & basil into another bowl & whisk thoroughly to combine
- Drizzle dressing over contents in the serving bowl & toss until well coated

Tasty Mediterranean Pilaf

Ingredients

1 small bell pepper

½ medium red onion

1 heaped tsp minced garlic

2 tsp rapeseed oil

1 large tomato

1 tbsp tomato paste

½ tsp ground cumin

¼ tsp ground cinnamon

Small pinch of salt

Small pinch of freshly ground black pepper

130g (drained weight) tinned chickpeas, rinsed with cold water

240ml low sodium vegetable stock

112g coarse bulgur wheat

Small pinch of chilli flakes

1 tbsp freshly chopped mint

1 tbsp chopped parsley

1 tbsp natural fat free yoghurt

6 olives

Instructions

- Deseed & chop pepper
- Dice onion & tomato
- Heat oil in a non-stick, lidded frying pan
- Add pepper, onion & garlic & stir-fry for 3 min, stirring frequently
- Mix in the tomato & fry for a further 2 min
- Add tomato paste, cumin, cinnamon, pinch of salt & pepper & mix well.
- Stir in chickpeas
- Add vegetable stock & bulgur wheat & stir thoroughly
- Cover & simmer mixture for 15 min or until bulgur wheat is cooked, adding a little water if longer cooking time is necessary
- Stir in chilli flakes, mint & parsley
- Remove from heat, cover & leave to rest for 5 min
- Spoon onto a plate
- Top with yoghurt & scatter olives on to serve

Rice Salad

Ingredients

70g short grain rice

½ small red onion

75g organic cucumber

30g grated carrot

1 tsp freshly grated ginger root

2 tbsp organic apple cider vinegar

2 tsp low sodium soy sauce

1 tsp sesame oil

2 tsp extra virgin olive oil

2 tsp sesame seeds

Instructions

- Cook rice following instructions on packet, drain, put into a serving bowl & leave until cooled
- Finely chop cucumber & onion

- Put cucumber, onion, grated carrot, grated ginger, vinegar, soy sauce, sesame oil & olive oil into another bowl & stir thoroughly until well mixed
- Spoon the above mixture over the rice & mix to combine
- Sprinkle with sesame seeds to serve

Stuffed Baked Sweet Potato

Ingredients

1 large sweet potato

2 tsp rapeseed oil

Handful of iceberg lettuce

½ medium onion

1 crushed garlic clove

4 cm of fresh ginger root

1 tsp curry paste of your choice

Pinch of freshly ground black pepper

1 tsp olive oil spread

60g baby spinach

6 cherry tomatoes

Instructions

- Preheat oven to 200^{0}C
- Use a fork to prick potato in several places
- Place potato on a foil-lined baking tray & brush with rapeseed oil if you want the skin to be crispy

- Bake potato for 1 hour or until soft inside when pierced with a sharp knife
- While it's baking make a bed of lettuce on a serving plate
- Finely chop the onion & grate the ginger
- Heat remaining oil in a non- stick frying pan
- Add onion & cook on medium-low heat until soft, approx 4 min, stirring often
- Add garlic & continue cooking for 1 min, stirring continuously
- Stir in curry paste, grated ginger & pepper & cook for 1 more min
- Add olive oil spread, reduce heat to low, add spinach & stir until it wilts, approx 1 min
- Place potato on a serving plate, slice open lengthwise & scoop out some of the soft flesh
- Remove frying pan from heat source & stir flesh into the curried mixture
- Spoon mixture carefully into potato, place on bed of lettuce & surround with tomatoes to serve

Simple Middle Eastern Dish

Ingredients

4 frozen falafels

60g dry couscous

2 medium vine tomatoes

75g organic cucumber

1 peeled medium carrot

Flesh of ½ small avocado

1 tbsp freshly squeezed lemon juice

2 tbsp hummus

A handful of rocket

1 tbsp edamame beans

1 tbsp freshly chopped coriander

1 tsp coriander seeds

Instructions

- Cook falafels & couscous following directions on the packs
- Meanwhile, on a large cutting board, chop tomatoes & cucumber, grate carrot & slice avocado
- Spoon hummus into a small bowl, stir in lemon juice & mix thoroughly to combine
- Scoop hummus onto centre of a serving plate
- Arrange rocket, tomato, cucumber, grated carrot, avocado slices & edamame beans around hummus leaving space for the falafel & couscous
- Add falafels & couscous
- Garnish contents of plate with fresh coriander & coriander seeds to complete

Vegetable Medley with Sweet Potato Mash

Ingredients

1 small onion

56g mushrooms

1 celery stalk

1 small carrot

1 parsnip

84g swede

1 medium-sized sweet potato

2 tsp rapeseed oil

250ml low sodium vegetable stock

¼ tsp yeast extract

1 tbsp tomato purée

6 cauliflower florets

½ tsp mixed herbs

1 bay leaf

½ tsp olive oil spread

1 tsp freshly chopped chives

Instructions

- Slice onion & mushrooms & chop celery, carrot, parsnip & swede

- Peel & chop sweet potato

- Heat oil in a non-stick lidded saucepan

- Add onion to saucepan & sauté until beginning to brown
- Pour in stock
- Add yeast extract & tomato purée & stir well until both dissolve
- Add celery, carrot, parsnip, swede, cauliflower, mushroom & half of the chopped potato
- Stir in mixed herbs & bay leaf
- Bring mixture to the boil on medium-high heat
- Reduce heat to low, cover & simmer gently for 20 min or until contents of pan are cooked, stirring occasionally
- Meanwhile, put the remaining chopped sweet potato into another saucepan, pour in water to cover potato, bring to the boil & cook for approx 15-20 min, until soft
- Drain potato, add spread & chives & mash in a bowl, with a fork
- Spoon mash onto the side of a dinner plate & ladle vegetable medley alongside it to serve

Quinoa with Egg, Beans & Tomato

Ingredients

56g quinoa

1 tsp extra virgin olive oil

Pinch of freshly ground black pepper

½ tsp organic apple cider vinegar

56g tinned black beans

1 tsp rapeseed oil

1 large free range egg

Flesh of ½ small avocado, sliced

6 cherry tomatoes cut into halves

1 tsp freshly chopped coriander

Instructions

- Rinse & cook quinoa according to instructions on packet

- While it's cooking, put olive oil, pepper & vinegar in a serving bowl & mix well
- Heat beans in their liquid in a saucepan, on low heat
- Drain & rinse beans, put into the bowl with quinoa & stir well
- Heat rapeseed oil in a non-stick frying pan on medium heat
- Fry egg to your satisfaction
- Transfer egg onto quinoa mixture
- Put avocado slices around the edge of the mixture with cherry tomatoes in between
- Sprinkle with coriander to serve

Wholewheat spaghetti with Tofu

Ingredients

75g wholewheat spaghetti

Olive oil cooking spray

1 tsp sesame oil

2½ cm of fresh ginger root

28g tinned water chestnuts, drained

84g tinned closed cup mushrooms, drained

2 crushed garlic cloves

2 tbsp low sodium soy sauce

150ml low sodium vegetable stock

1 tsp chickpea flour

56g trimmed asparagus spears

56g firm tofu

Instructions

- Cook spaghetti according to instructions on packet

- Meanwhile, chop ginger & water chestnuts
- Drain & press tofu between paper towelling, then chop finely
- Spray a large non-stick saucepan with cooking spray
- Add sesame oil & heat on low
- Add ginger & garlic & cook for 3 min, stirring frequently
- Stir in soy sauce & half the stock
- Cook for 5 min on medium heat
- Mix rest of stock with chickpea flour until smooth then add to pan, lower heat & simmer, stirring continuously, until sauce thickens, approx 3 min
- Add asparagus, water chestnuts, mushrooms & tofu
- Cook contents of pan for 3 min longer
- Drain cooked spaghetti & stir into the sauce
- Serve in a bowl while hot

Courgettes & Onion with Wholewheat Spaghetti

Ingredients

75g wholewheat spaghetti

Olive oil cooking spray

1 medium courgette, thickly sliced

½ medium onion, thickly sliced

½ tsp freshly ground black pepper

1½ tbsp grated Emmental cheese

1 tbsp freshly chopped parsley

Bowl of mixed green salad of your choice

Dressing for salad

2 tsp extra virgin olive oil

1 tsp organic apple cider vinegar

1 tsp wholegrain mustard

Small pinch of freshly chopped basil

Instructions

- Preheat oven to 240^{0}C
- Meanwhile, cut courgette & onion into thick slices
- Put spaghetti on to cook following instructions on packet
- Spread courgette & onion slices onto a large foil-lined baking tray & spray lightly with oil to coat thoroughly
- Put dressing ingredients into a small bowl & mix well
- Bake courgette & onion for 8-10 min or until veg is tender on the inside but crisp outside
- Drain spaghetti & tip into a serving bowl
- Mix courgette & onion into spaghetti
- Sprinkle with cheese & garnish with parsley
- Pour dressing over your mixed green salad, toss to coat & serve with the spaghetti mixture

Easy Beany Egg

Ingredients

2 tsp rapeseed oil

1 small onion

1 clove of garlic

130g (drained weight) tinned cannellini beans, rinsed

with cold water

¼ tsp ground paprika

227g tinned chopped tomatoes

1 tbsp freshly chopped chives

Pinch of freshly ground black pepper

1 heaped tsp freshly chopped flat parsley

1 large free range egg

Instructions

- Dice onion & cut garlic into thin slices

- Heat oil in a non-stick, lidded fry pan on medium heat

- Stir diced onion & garlic slices into oil & cook for 3

  min, stirring frequently

- Stir in paprika, tomatoes, chives, black pepper & parsley

- Cook, stirring continuously, for 2 min

- Add beans, mix well & simmer for 2 further min

- Make a space in the middle of the beany mixture & crack egg into it

- Cover pan & cook for 2-4 min, until the egg is cooked as you like it

- Transfer contents of pan carefully onto a serving plate & enjoy

Nut Roast with Cauliflower, Carrot & Peas

Ingredients

½ small onion

½ small clove garlic

2 tsp rapeseed oil

17g fine wholemeal breadcrumbs

37g ground mixed nuts

40ml low sodium vegetable stock

1 tsp soy sauce

½ tsp dried herbs

½ tsp chia seeds

3 florets cauliflower

1 medium-sized sliced carrot

1 tbsp frozen garden peas

Instructions

- Preheat the oven to 200^0C

- Dice onion & finely chop garlic

- Heat oil in a small non-stick frying pan over medium-low heat

- Sauté onion & garlic for about 3 min or until soft & translucent

- Put onion & garlic into a bowl

- Stir in breadcrumbs, nuts, stock, soy sauce, chia seeds & dried herbs

- Grease a small (7.5-9cm) ramekin & line base with greaseproof paper

- Spoon the mixture from the bowl into the ramekin

- Roast in the oven for 20 min or until the top of your roast has a golden brown crust

- Steam cauliflower & carrots over a pan of boiling water for approx 10 min or until just tender

- Remove ramekin from oven & allow to stand for five min to enable the roast to become firm

- Meanwhile, put peas into a small microwavable bowl with 2 tsp water & microwave for 1 min, depending on your microwave wattage, then drain them

- Turn your roast onto a plate & serve with cauliflower, carrot & peas

Filled Mushrooms Topped with Feta & Chives

Ingredients

3 large mushrooms with stems removed

1 tsp extra virgin olive oil

1 tbsp chopped yellow pepper

1 tsp chopped green olives

1 heaped tsp finely chopped parsley

1 tbsp chopped cherry tomatoes

½ medium-sized crushed garlic clove

¼ tsp freshly chopped oregano

¼ tsp freshly squeezed lemon juice

Freshly ground black pepper, to taste

28g feta cheese

1 tbsp freshly chopped chives

Instructions

- Heat oven to 190°C
- Place mushrooms on a foil-lined baking tray

- Put oil, yellow pepper, olives, parsley, tomatoes, garlic, oregano, lemon juice & black pepper into a bowl & mix together thoroughly
- Spoon the mix from the bowl equally into each mushroom
- Bake for 20 min
- Transfer filled mushrooms to a plate, crumble feta cheese & sprinkle over
- Top each mushroom with chives before serving